CAUSES AND HOW TO STOP PREGNANCY LOSS

A brief guide for understanding and addressing pregnancy miscarriage

Julius Abdul

s

Disclaimer

This book is for informational purposes only and is not intended to be a substitute for professional medical advice, diagnosis, or treatment. Always seek the advice of your physician with any questions you may have regarding a medical condition. Always consult with your physician before starting any exercise program or doing anything contained in this book. Always stop if you experience any pain, discomfort, or difficulties performing anything described in this book.

Table of Content

Introduction   7

Figure Out Why   10

Test Don't Guess   12

Evaluation   15

Diet   17

Toxics   19

Lifestyle   21

Support   23

Conclusion   25

Introduction

Pregnancy is a journey filled with hope, anticipation, and dreams of the future. However, for many, this path can be fraught with heartache and loss. Miscarriage and stillbirth are profound tragedies that affect countless families, leaving emotional scars that are often difficult to heal.

It's hard, painful, and heart-wrenching because you've got your hopes up this whole time thinking everything will be great, and in the end, it wasn't. And on top of it, it potentially makes the next time you get pregnant even harder emotionally because you're scared every week that you go on that something is going to happen. The only positive thing that comes from a miscarriage is that the first step in getting to a healthy pregnancy is achieved. The fact that you have been able to get pregnant in the past, moving forward, doesn't explain why you haven't been able to hold a pregnancy which will lead to the loss of hope that you're going to be able to hold a pregnancy in the future. This book is designed to support those navigating these challenging waters, offering evidence-based strategies, compassionate advice, and practical tools to help prevent pregnancy loss.

Pregnancy loss and miscarriage are some of the most frequent cases in hospitals and clinics that are attended to daily, fortunately, there is so much that can be done which will be covered in this book.

Whether you've had one miscarriage or none at all, there are potential things that you can do to avoid that risk in the future and for future pregnancies. One big fact that is important for us to know is that about 80% of all miscarriages occur in the first trimester.

What defines the first trimester? Most people think that the first trimester is up until 12 weeks, but the reality is, if you've been pregnant before and you know how you start to calculate your pregnancy, you'll realize that most people calculate their pregnancies from the date of their last period. That's right, because we all know you were not pregnant at your period of menstruation, but will conceive two weeks later at ovulation, hopefully.

Therefore, two weeks is added to the calculation process making it easier to calculate a pregnancy from the date of your last period because that's a known quantity than some other time when we're not quite sure where exactly you ovulated. this is why two other weeks are added to the calculation taking the first trimester to 14 weeks, and, that's done in many other countries as well. Regardless, the statistics for pregnancy loss and miscarriage are calculated at 12 weeks, and the likelihood of having a loss after 12 weeks goes down considerably. So that's why it's important to understand where you are in the pregnancy and how important this first trimester is to maintaining a healthy pregnancy. We put so much emphasis on the first trimester for this reason, and it's not to say that you can't have a loss beyond the first trimester, that those are less likely. This book will be focused on this first piece, this first-trimester portion of things.

Your reproductive system is not the most vital in the body, and as such, it takes a backseat when other things start to go wrong or go off and your body's not functioning optimally. when something is going on in the body and it's not functioning properly, it will allocate appropriate resources to that part of the body or that system to get it back on track. And as such, it puts your reproductive function and holding a pregnancy on the back burner.

It will be like, "You know what? This is not so important right now, and so we're not going to make this the most important thing. We're going to prioritize what's important for your health and ssafety and staying alive, and we're going to focus on those things right now." And when that happens, the body is not functioning at a hundred percent, so in turn, the body says, "Well, we need to do something about this. It's not safe to hold a pregnancy or it's not safe to get pregnant." And what ends up happening over time is that in dealing with the area, the system, issue, or disease that's going on, the body is prioritizing that, and it ends up over time, having a miscarriage or your immune system is not supporting that because it's focusing on something else, and again, you have a loss. And this is exactly what we're trying to prevent. We're trying to understand what function is not happening properly, why that's not happening, and give the body the support that it needs so that body can go back to homeostasis and balance to give the appropriate resources that it needs to not only getting pregnant but maintaining a healthy pregnancy.

First things first, when something is going on, we need to figure out why, So the first chapter of this book is to figure out why.

Figure Out Why

It is super important to know the possible causes and reasons why you might be having a loss. I know that might seem either simple or complex, but this should be your first place of consideration, so you are recommended to take a step back, and take inventory of your body, your health, your environment, and your life, and start to write down the areas that you would like to see improved. These are things that you should know. I mean, maybe you know that you just need more energy, Let's keep it simple, you're not sleeping enough or not well, maybe you need to eat better. In the process of taking note of all these, I want you to be as broad as you can, also considering your emotions, stress, or maybe work, whatever it might be, you need to take inventory so that we can start to unravel the possible causes or influences that might be impacting your ability to hold on and have a healthy pregnancy.

The next chapter of this book is connected to this because It urges you to, "test, don't guess."

Summary

The chapter emphasizes the importance of identifying possible causes for any issues you might be experiencing, particularly in relation to maintaining a healthy pregnancy. It advises taking a step back to assess various aspects of your life, including your body, health, environment, and lifestyle. By doing so, you should note areas needing improvement, such as sleep quality, diet, energy levels, and emotional well-being. A comprehensive inventory, considering factors like stress and work, will help identify influences affecting your ability to sustain a healthy pregnancy.

Test Don't Guess

This is connected to the previous discussion because we're trying to find out the underlying causes. So in addition to you taking inventory in step number one, we also want you to do some testing, or additional labs testing so that we can start to put what you took in from number one, your medical history, which I'm going to label as number two, and what we're doing right now in number two which is testing, and putting all of that together to start to create your picture to understand why you might be having the losses that you've had or been having. So, when we start or continue on this test piece and want to do some additional testing, the first two things that are essential to test are the immune function and your blood clotting factors. Those are the two most common reasons why you might be having a pregnancy loss.

The third common reason is genetic testing. There are additional tests that you can do to look at the genetic side of things to see if any of those are potentially contributing to the losses as well.

Another recommended test that should be done, and these are all potential reasons that could be contributing to a miscarriage or pregnancy loss, is thyroid function. considering a full thyroid panel, because having an autoimmune thyroid, which would be classified under autoimmune testing or immune testing, and proper thyroid function can impact your ability to hold a pregnancy.

Egg quality can certainly do it. I don't think it's as common as we say it is or think or believe that it is, but certainly egg quality, if egg quality is compromised, it could lead to a miscarriage. Sperm quality is the same. We forget or don't believe that sperm can contribute to pregnancy loss. But absolutely, 40 to 50% of all miscarriages can be attributed in some way to a male factor or sperm quality issue.

Two other areas that we need to rule out here, are PCOS, and polycystic ovarian syndrome. When you do all your initial testing, you should have already ruled this out, but if not, then we need to include that in the testing, because if you have polycystic ovarian syndrome, then you are more likely to have a miscarriage as well. And then obesity, which may or may not need additional testing, but certainly doing a "Body Mass Index" (BMI), because the higher your BMI, the more likely you are to have a loss. So those are the bigger pieces, the bigger places that we want to do more investigation and testing as part of this chapter.

The third chapter is still in this evaluation and assessment phase, whether it's lab or otherwise, we have to evaluate and look.

Summary

"Test Don't Guess," is focus on the importance of comprehensive testing to identify the underlying causes of pregnancy loss. The process begins with taking an inventory of your medical history. Additional testing is recommended to piece together a complete picture of why pregnancy losses might be occurring.
Key tests to consider include:
1. Immune Function: Testing for immune issues is critical as they are a common cause of pregnancy loss.
2. Blood Clotting Factors: Abnormalities in blood clotting can lead to miscarriages.
3. Genetic Testing: This helps identify any genetic factors that might contribute to pregnancy loss.
4. Thyroid Function: A full thyroid panel is essential because thyroid issues, including autoimmune thyroid conditions, can impact pregnancy.
5. Egg and Sperm Quality: Both egg and sperm quality should be evaluated, as issues here can lead to

miscarriages. Male factors contribute to 40-50% of miscarriages.

6. PCOS (Polycystic Ovarian Syndrome): This should be ruled out as it increases the risk of miscarriage.

7. Obesity: A high Body Mass Index *(BMI) can increase the likelihood of pregnancy loss.*

These tests are crucial in understanding the various factors that might be contributing to pregnancy losses, enabling a more targeted and effective approach to prevention and treatment.

Evaluation

Other systems of the body can also impact your ability to get and stay pregnant, so, we will want to look at: What is going on in your digestive system? What is going on in your pelvic area with the uterus? These are all potential reasons that could also contribute to a loss, and these are things that we tend to look at much later. If after these investigations there is still a loss, we will then start looking for maybe some of those more uncommon or obscure reasons like digestive issues. Relative records and research have proven that digestive issues can also contribute to pregnancy loss, and so we want to make sure we evaluate that.

The best way to start evaluating that is through stool testing. And then there's more advanced testing where we're looking at the tissue from the uterus or the endometrium, and those are biopsied or taken out and sent for testing because you're looking for any abnormal bacteria, infections, inflammation, endometriosis, and so forth. So those are all part of this well-rounded approach to get a better understanding of what's going on with your body so that it can be addressed for a future positive impact.

The next important step that will need our attention is our diet.

summary

In the chapter "Evaluation," the highlights is on the importance of examining various body systems that can affect pregnancy. Beyond the primary tests, attention should also be given to the digestive system and pelvic area, including the uterus. These areas are often overlooked but can contribute to pregnancy loss.
Key points include:
1. Digestive System: Digestive issues can impact pregnancy, and stool testing is a primary method for evaluation.
2. Pelvic Area and Uterus: Advanced testing, such as biopsies of uterine or endometrial tissue, can identify abnormal bacteria, infections, inflammation, or conditions like endometriosis.
This comprehensive approach ensures a thorough understanding of the body's potential issues, aiding in the prevention and treatment of pregnancy loss for future positive outcomes.

Diet

Remember you are recommended to take inventory of your overall life and what might need to be improved, diet was one of the things we mentioned, but it also needs time for itself. It needs a separate section when taking these inventories because oftentimes we don't put enough energy into this. Even though we know we should be doing better with it, we don't, because we have certain cravings and desires and it is hard to break, it's difficult to change our diet.

Your diet is super important. Not only is it important just because we want you to eat healthy, but if we find out that there are issues, let's just say with immune function or blood clotting variables or polycystic ovarian syndrome or whatever it might be, those conditions will impact your diet and your diet will impact those conditions. So, we need to make sure that you're eating appropriately based on our findings. For now, there will not be specific suggestions, but once we know what your findings are and why you're having these issues, then that's where we come back and have a more tailored specific approach to your diet. But right here, you just need to know how important it is and why we at least need to at the bare minimum, clean it up, eat whole foods, and get rid of processed foods, sugars, and all the junk food that we know is just not good for us. Those are things that you can start doing to clean up your diet.

Toxins should be removed especially those pesky, dirty toxins that we are exposed to regularly.

summary

This chapter "Diet," unveils the significance of diet in the broader context of understanding and addressing pregnancy loss. While taking an inventory of your overall life, diet merits special attention due to its profound impact on health.

Key points include:

1. Importance of Diet: Diet plays a crucial role not only for general health but also in managing specific conditions that could affect pregnancy, such as immune function, blood clotting disorders, and PCOS.
2. Challenges in Changing Diet: Acknowledging the difficulty in changing dietary habits due to cravings and desires, the chapter stresses the need for commitment to improvement.

3. Interrelationship with Health Conditions: Diet can influence and be influenced by health conditions, making it essential to tailor dietary recommendations based on specific findings related to pregnancy loss.

4. Initial Steps for Improvement: While specific dietary suggestions will come after identifying the underlying causes, the chapter advises starting with general improvements. This includes eating whole foods and eliminating processed foods, sugars, and junk food.

The overarching message is that a clean, healthy diet is foundational and can significantly impact the ability to address and manage factors contributing to pregnancy loss.

Toxics

This is an important topic that will increase our overall wellness when properly understood, it has a long way effect when it comes to fertility if properly addressed. Getting rid of toxins has a way of cleaning things up which will improve the body's function and as well the sperm quality. People who are passing through this phase usually give information on their diet and environment and then ask their fertility coaches or doctors for feedback.

You have to be reasonable about this, bearing in mind that the suggestions in terms of cleaning things up are going to be focused on removing as much toxin exposure and reducing chemical toxin load as possible. This is something that needs to happen throughout our lives because we're exposed to toxins and chemicals in many ways.

But one of the main areas that I think is important for us to talk about is Roundup. Now Glyphosate is found in so much of our food supply, and the places that we don't think it is are the places it's probably found the most. If you're drinking coffee, it is always advised to drink organic coffee if you must have coffee, it's because all these pesticides and toxins are sprayed heavily on those coffee beans. We want to eliminate that as much as possible.

We also find it in all the alcohol, especially the main ones that you consume. All beer, and all wine from the United States, you bet, has a ton of pesticides and Roundup in it, even the organic ones because they can't avoid it, the reason being is that most people have one organic plot in the middle of conventional farming around them, and all of that seeps into the water, gets passed into the air, and still lands in that area. So, they might have less, but they still have it.

Beer and wine in my mind are a no-no, if you're going to be consuming alcohol. I just suggest you just avoid beer altogether because we just don't know how to manage that.

We want to eliminate toxins from every part of our lives as much as we can control, and that's something that should last a lifetime. This cannot be overemphasized how important it is to take notes.

summary

The chapter "Toxics" talked about the significant impact of toxin exposure on overall wellness and fertility. Properly addressing toxins can enhance body function and sperm quality.

Key points include:

1. Diet and Environment: Individuals should provide detailed information on their diet and environmental exposures to their fertility coaches or doctors for personalized feedback.
2. Reducing Toxin Exposure: Focus on minimizing exposure to toxins and chemicals. This is a lifelong effort as toxins are ubiquitous.
3. Glyphosate (Roundup: Found in many foods, particularly in non-organic coffee, beer, and wine. Even organic options can be contaminated due to proximity to conventional farming.
4. Organic Choices: Opt for organic coffee and avoid alcohol, especially beer, due to high levels of pesticides and glyphosate.

By reducing toxin exposure, one can significantly improve fertility and overall health.

Lifestyle

Review your lifestyle habits. That's right. What in your lifestyle could you improve, that is also going to help you not only get pregnant, but stay pregnant, Managing your stress is number one, because managing our stress, especially while we're going through a miscarriage or after a miscarriage, but especially once we get pregnant because it's difficult to not start to worry and think about if this pregnancy is going to last, there are applications like FertileMind app that can do wonders for you and your anxiety and stress moving forward. It's going to help you manage all of that so that it can be easier to hopefully get pregnant and stay pregnant.

The next thing to concentrate on could potentially be the most important piece, which is to: Seek out additional help and support so that you can get the right support that you need.

Summary

In the chapter "Lifestyle," the highlights are on the importance of reviewing and improving lifestyle habits to enhance the chances of getting and staying pregnant. The primary focus is on managing stress, especially during and after a miscarriage, and once pregnant. Managing stress is crucial as it helps reduce anxiety and worry about the pregnancy's viability. The author recommends using tools like the FertileMind app, which can help manage anxiety and stress, thereby supporting better pregnancy outcomes.

Support

This could be the missing piece because it's so hard to put all the other pieces in order of priority and it's even hard to get all the testing done without getting the proper support that you need. Are you getting the proper support? Are they thinking about your losses and making those a priority for you? Are they looking and investigating in the right place? Most of these patients attending clinic and hospital check always say the same thing, they often say, my doctor said at the next loss, we can look at those things, or It's not important right now, we're fine for it now, but if it happens again, we can investigate. Why do we want a loss again? Why not start investigating now? I mean, maybe we're not doing all the testing that I recommended, but why not start to dig now so that you can have at least some peace of mind that you're being proactive, that your doctor is also being proactive, and you are starting to look in the areas that need to be looked at, having it in mind that you deserve all that.

You need to get proper support, not only for the investigation of the right areas, but it will also help to have the necessary information available to create the appropriate plan to address your needs, which is super important and key.

summary

In the chapter "Support," the author highlights the critical role of proper support in managing pregnancy loss. It is challenging to prioritize and complete all necessary tests without adequate support. The key questions to consider are:
- Are you receiving the proper support?
- Is your support system prioritizing your pregnancy losses?
- Are they investigating the right areas?
Patients often hear from doctors that investigations can wait until another loss occurs. However, this approach can lead to repeated heartbreak and frustration. The author advocates for proactive investigation and support now, rather than waiting for another loss. Even if not all recommended tests are performed immediately, starting some investigations can provide peace of mind and demonstrate a proactive approach from both the patient and the doctor.
Proper support is essential not only for investigating the right areas but also for gathering the necessary information

to create an appropriate plan to address individual needs. This proactive and supportive approach is key to addressing pregnancy loss effectively.

Conclusion

Pregnancy loss is a deeply challenging and often misunderstood experience. This book has aimed to shed light on the multifaceted causes and potential solutions for those who face this heart-wrenching journey. By focusing on key areas such as medical history, immune function, blood clotting factors, genetic testing, thyroid function, egg and sperm quality, PCOS, and obesity, we have explored the various factors that can contribute to pregnancy loss.

The importance of diet, toxin exposure, and lifestyle habits has been emphasized as critical components that impact fertility and pregnancy outcomes. Understanding these aspects allows individuals to take control of their health and make informed decisions that can improve their chances of a successful pregnancy.

A significant takeaway is the need for comprehensive testing and the proactive investigation of potential issues. "Test, Don't Guess" underscores the value of thorough testing to identify and address the root causes of pregnancy loss, rather than relying on assumptions or waiting for repeated losses to prompt action.

Equally crucial is the support system surrounding those experiencing pregnancy loss. The chapter on "Support" highlights the necessity of having a dedicated and proactive medical team that prioritizes investigating and addressing pregnancy loss. Patients deserve to have their concerns taken seriously and to receive the necessary support to navigate this difficult journey.

In summary, the path to understanding and addressing pregnancy loss is complex and multifaceted. By prioritizing comprehensive testing, adopting a proactive and informed approach, and ensuring robust support systems, individuals can better understand the underlying causes of pregnancy loss and work towards successful pregnancies. This book serves as a guide to empower individuals with the knowledge and tools needed to take charge of their reproductive health and move forward with hope and confidence.